SKINCARE SECRETS FROM THE
INSIDE OUT

A STEP BY STEP GUIDE TO
GREAT SKIN AT ANY AGE

DR. LAURA ELLIS, MD

TABLE OF CONTENTS

FOREWORD 5

PART I—BEAUTIFUL, HEALTHY, VIBRANT SKIN... *FROM THE INSIDE OUT* 7

PART II—ANTI-AGING THERAPIES FOR SKIN THAT STANDS THE TEST OF TIME 13

PART III—COLD SORE PREVENTION & IMMUNE SYSTEM SUPPORT 18

FAQs 23

FOREWORD

Welcome to beautiful, blemish-free skin! In this booklet I am pleased to share with you my secrets to healthy, radiant, ageless skin.

Having passed the 50-year mark, I am flattered when my patients compliment me on my skin. Frequently I'm asked how I take care of my skin and make it glow and look so healthy. So, I'm finally putting it all down in writing for you!

I was not one of those people born with beautiful skin. When I was a teen, my skin was a mess. It was uncontrollably oily and blemished. In those days, there were few good remedies for difficult teenage skin. My doctor recommended a harsh scrub with sulfur and salicylic acid that caused terrible dryness and cracking. I was afraid moisturizers would only make the situation worse. Fortunately, a friend's mother recognized my problem and showed me a better way. A gentle cleanser and light moisturizer were all it took to turn things around. Just those two small changes made a huge difference! And, when I left home for college and taught myself how to shop for and prepare nutritious meals, my skin improved even more!

Ever since that pivotal time, skin care has been an important part of my day. For more than 35 years I've followed a ritual of healthy living and dedicated skin care. A degree in Biochemistry gave me a sound scientific foundation in nutrition and metabolism, while my experience working with thousands of patients gave me a practical understanding of the problems people struggle with most. After finding ways to heal myself, I felt a deep passion to share what I'd learned with others.

Anyone who has suffered from acne or other skin problems knows the toll it can take on your self-esteem. It can make you self-conscious and uncomfortable around other people, no matter what your age. No one should suffer this way! Let me assure you that even if you haven't always practiced the healthiest lifestyle, it's never too late to start. Our bodies have an amazing ability to repair and restore. Start now, and you will soon be pleased with the healthy, radiant face that looks back at you in the mirror!

Let's take a look inside together—because beautiful, blemish-free skin starts *from the Inside Out.*

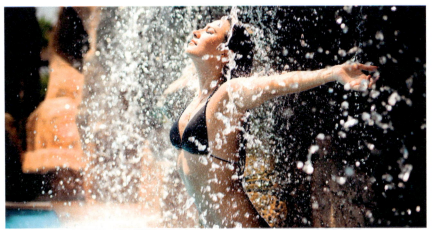

PART I—BEAUTIFUL, HEALTHY, VIBRANT SKIN... *FROM THE INSIDE OUT*

They say that beauty is only skin deep, but the truth is that beautiful, radiant skin starts deep within. What we take into our bodies is critical to how our skin looks on the outside. We all know that if we eat fatty, sugary foods our bodies will begin to change shape and it becomes much more challenging to get back to our ideal weight. The same is true of our skin. Maintaining our complexion through healthy daily rituals and nurturing attention will ensure that it is ageless and resilient through all the stages of our lives.

So let's begin from the most important place... *from the inside out.*

HOW DOES OUR SKIN WORK?
The main function of our skin is to act as a physical, chemical, and antibacterial defense system. If we work with our skin instead of against it, our skin has natural rejuvenating and reparative properties.

The top layer of our skin, called the stratum corneum, helps to limit the loss of water (moisture) and protects against external toxins, such as chemicals and bacteria. Stratum corneum cells originate in the deep layers of the epidermis and migrate toward the surface, shedding in 4–6 weeks. This process of producing new cells and replacing old ones is continuous and natural... but it is not always perfect.

THINGS THAT INTERFERE WITH NATURAL SKIN REJUVENATION
A number of factors can break down the barrier of the stratum corneum, compromising the proper function of enzymes that naturally loosen the bonds between skin cells and allow shedding of them one at a time. These include:

- Daily damage from poor cleansers
- Too frequent or too rigorous cleansings
- Low humidity
- Wind and UV light
- Stress
- Dehydration

TELLTALE SIGNS OF DYSFUNCTIONAL SKIN
Our skin is a good reflection of what is going on inside us. It can reveal the imbalances in our lives, whether physical or emotional.

- It is rough and dull looking.
- It is pale rather than pink and glowing.
- It may show visible signs of scaling and cracking.
- It may show premature fine lines that are not a natural part of aging.
- It looks uneven, with no consistency in tone.
- It doesn't snap back when pinched.

GET STARTED AND GO NATURAL
As your largest organ, your skin needs a lot of attention. But this needn't be burdensome or time-consuming. Make your skin rituals as automatic as brushing your teeth or taking your daily multivitamin. As long as it is well hydrated and supported by good lifestyle habits, your skin is remarkably efficient at repairing itself without the need for chemical peels, laser treatments or cosmeceuticals.

GUT INSTINCTS
The ability to absorb nutrients from our foods, to digest them well, and then to eliminate them regularly is critical to healthy skin. Everyone knows the link between constipation and breakouts. To facilitate optimal bioabsorption and proper digestion, it is necessary to build a colony of healthy bacteria (microflora) in the gut. This "good bacteria" builds energy, strengthens our immunity, and promotes detoxification. A healthy "Mediterranean" diet that is vegetable-based, high in healthy fats and proteins, low in processed foods and sugars, and includes probiotics, e.g. yogurt, kefir, and sauerkraut, is critical to a healthy gut and, in turn, to healthy, vibrant skin.

You may have heard of "leaky gut," which refers to intestinal permeability resulting in inflammation and poor nutritional intake. But we also have what might be called "leaky skin." Research has shown that stress and inflammation caused by gut imbalances can compromise the skin's ability to protect and repair itself.

DIET
Just as with your body, your skin prefers whole, pure, organic foods.

SKIN HEALTHY FOODS
- Avocados
- Healthy oils (olive, flaxseed, coconut)
- Green tea
- Dark, leafy greens (kale, spinach, arugula, etc.)
- Berries (blueberries, raspberries, blackberries, etc.)
- Seeds (flax, pumpkin, sunflower, etc.)

- Carotene-rich foods such as sweet potatoes, pumpkin, carrots
- Probiotics such as sugar free yogurt and cultured vegetables
- Quinoa and other low-glycemic grains
- Mineral-rich foods like sea vegetables
- Omega-3 fatty acids (found in fatty fish like salmon, tuna, sardines)
- Healthy herbs like rosemary, thyme, basil, and oregano

FOODS TO AVOID
- Greasy, fatty, fried foods that are difficult to digest
- Foods high in refined carbohydrates, such as chips, pretzels, white rice and pasta
- Packaged and highly processed foods, such as most takeout or prepackaged dinners
- Foods high in white sugar, fructose, and corn syrup

MYTH:
Chocolate doesn't make your face break out. If you notice breakouts around the time of your menstrual cycle, you may wrongly assume that your chocolate craving is to blame. In fact, it is just normal hormone fluctuations, particularly in progesterone, which cause an increase in facial oils, such as sebum, that build up in our pores and cause acne. In fact, dark chocolate contains anti-aging antioxidants called flavonoids, which fight free radicals to protect skin from UV damage and help prevent the appearance of wrinkles, fine lines, and skin discolorations.

FOODS TO LIMIT
The foods listed below are not unhealthy when consumed in moderation, but for some people, they may lead to skin problems.
- Foods high in citric acid
- High fat foods such as butter and cream
- Coffee or other high-caffeine beverages
- Gluten-heavy grains
- Alcohol (especially mixed drinks. Wine is better, but stick with red.)
- Milk (especially if it is not organic. Try almond, coconut or kefir milk as alternatives.)

HYDRATION
It's critical to drink pure water throughout the day. Most of us drink water only when our mouths get dry, and we can be systemically dehydrated without knowing it. As we get older, we become even less aware of when we're thirsty, and can go for longer periods without perceiving thirst. For this reason we need to be very conscientious about our water intake. (Some people even set alarms to alert them when it's time for a water break.)

Most of us are chronically dehydrated, which limits proper cellular enzymatic function. This can lead to moodiness and poor concentration, neuromuscular disability and, in the case of wrinkles, poor detachment of naturally shedding skin cells. When we are chronically dehydrated our skin cells will shed in clumps rather than cell by cell. Clump shedding is why skin can look "dull" instead of bright and becoming.

The standard recommendation for daily water intake is to drink half of your body weight in ounces, so if you weigh 200 pounds that would mean at least four 12-oz. glasses a day. But please realize that your hydration needs can vary based on your level of physical activity, health conditions and medications, and the climate in which you live. The best waters are those from natural mineral springs, ideally high in silica (Si), as well as being alkaline, such as Fiji, Volvic, New Zealand, and 1907. Silica is important for the formation and optimal maintenance of collagen. Another benefit is that it is a natural chelator of the heavy metal aluminum (Al). This metal not only plays havoc with your skin by binding to collagen and altering protein metabolism, but it's even harder on your brain. In fact, high Al levels in drinking waters in areas around the world have a higher correlation with Alzheimer's and other types of cognitive impairment.

Hydration is also about using an effective moisturizer that contains a good humectant (moisture preserver), such as glycerol, to hold water in, as well as lipid emollients that seal in moisture and prevent washout of the humectant when the skin is in contact with water.

DAILY CLEANSING RITUALS

EVERYDAY CLEANSING - To prevent water loss through the skin, the natural moisture barrier must not be stripped away with overly rigorous cleansing or harsh products.

For daily cleansing, use a non-abrasive, non-soap cleanser (such as Neutrogena or Cetaphil), washing and then towel drying the skin gently. This should be followed by application of an eye cream and a moisturizer to the face, neck and décolleté area to protect the natural moisture barrier. If your skin is on the sebaceous (oily) side, I recommend a non-soap cleanser that contains 1–2% salicylic acid, which helps to unplug blocked skin pores and soften and loosen dry skin so that it falls off more easily.

TWICE A WEEK - Every few days modify this routine slightly by gently exfoliating the skin with a washcloth to remove accumulated dead skin, dirt and makeup. Please note: vigorous scrubbing of the skin can aggravate an existing skin condition and deplete the skin of its natural moisturizing oils.

AT NIGHT - One of the worst things you can do for your skin is to go to bed without washing your face. When you go to sleep with makeup and other impurities on your face, it is much more likely that you'll be staring at a breakout the next morning. After gentle cleansing and/or exfoliating, make sure you apply an overnight moisturizer to your face before bedtime. If you are someone who enjoys baths in the evenings, there are some very gentle exfoliating scrubs that help to slough off dead skin cells and boost circulation, leaving your skin smooth and well moisturized. (Note: use these just on the body, as they may be too abrasive for the face.)

See page 11 for a list of recommended cleansers, moisturizers, body exfoliants, and sunscreens.

CRITICAL LIFESTYLE FACTORS
- **STRESS MANAGEMENT** - Psychological stress has been tied to a long list of health issues, including skin problems. A study in The Journal of Clinical Investigation showed that psychological stress disrupts the skin's antimicrobial barrier. Find ways to be good to yourself throughout the day. Take short "mental health" breaks and find some time for activities that are calming, whether it is a gentle yoga class, meditating or drawing. Avoid people who raise your anxiety levels and resist the expectations of perfection.
- **SLEEP** - Lack of sleep alters cortisol levels, creates stress and weakens the adrenals. Most sleep experts recommend between 7 and 8 hours of regular sleep each night. That means each and every night. When we sleep our skin does most of its repair work, creating new cells and shedding and repairing old and damaged ones.

- **EXERCISE** - Daily exercise that stimulates circulation, massages the lymph glands, and promotes detoxification through sweating is critical for healthy skin. Nothing beats exercise for brightening the eyes and putting roses in the cheeks. Exercise also tightens and tones the skin. Be sure to always hydrate well before and afterwards.

- **NO SMOKING** - Smoking destroys the tiny arteries that sustain your skin. It has long been associated with premature aging—showing up in fine lines around the mouth and eyes.

- **NO TANNING** - The sun's ultraviolet radiation (UVR) is the cause of most skin cancers, many cataracts and 90% of visible aging. While it is important for bone and skin health to get plenty of Vitamin D, it is a myth that you can get enough Vitamin D with just 15 minutes of sun everyday. It is important to protect the skin from over-exposure ultraviolet rays. Never sit in the sun to the point of sunburn and always wear a sunscreen, not just in the summer months, but year round.

SOME THINGS TO REMEMBER ABOUT UVR:
- UVR is strongest between 10:00 AM and 2:00 PM.
- Clouds filter some, but not most, of the UVR, so it's still possible to get burned on a cloudy day.
- UVA rays pass through windows (even car windows).
- UVA rays penetrate deep into the dermis, (lower layer of skin), causing DNA and collagen damage.
- Some ground surfaces such as sand and snow reflect most of the UVR. For instance, snow can reflect as much as 80% of the incident UVR.
- Water actually reflects very little UVR.
- For every 1000 feet increase in altitude the UVR increases by 4%.

> Now that you know the basics of beautiful skin, I'd like to share with you some of the common skin problems my clients struggle with, including those that are specific to aging. I'll also talk a bit more about clinically effective anti-aging therapies that will keep your skin vibrant and healthy throughout the years.

YOUR INSIDE OUT SHOPPING LIST

CLEANSERS

FOR OILY, SENSITIVE SKIN:
$ Aveeno Clear Complexion Foaming Cleanser
$ Neutrogena Oil-Free Acne Wash
$$ Topix Clay Sal 5-2 Cleanser
$$$ Vivite Exfoliating Facial Cleanser

FOR DRYER SKIN:
$ Cera Ve Hydrating Cleanser
$ Aveeno Positively Radiant Cleanser
$$ Nia 24 Physical Cleansing Scrub
$$ Murad Essential-C Cleanser

MOISTURIZERS

DAY-TIME
1. $ Aveeno Ultra-Calming Daily Moisture SPF 15
2. $ Cetaphil Daily Facial Moisturizer SPF 15
3. $ Purpose Dual Treatment Moisture Lotion SPF 15
4. $$ SkinCeuticals Daily Sun Defense SPF 20
5. $$$ Nia24 Sun Damage Prevention 100% Mineral Sunscreen

BED-TIME
1. $ Aveeno Ultra-Calming Moisturizing Cream
2. $$ Burt's Bees Evening Primrose Overnight Cream
3. $$ Elizabeth Arden Good Night's Sleep Restoring Cream
4. $$ La Roche-Posay Toleriane Soothing Protective Facial Cream
5. $$$ Bobbi Brown Intensive Skin Supplement

BODY EXFOLIANTS

1. $ Exfoliating shower glove and cloth
2. $$ Hempz Age Defying Glycolic Herbal Body Scrub with light glycolic acid
3. $$$ PCA Body Therapy with 12% Lactic acid

UV PROTECTION/SUNSCREENS

1. $$ PCA Weightless Protection Broad Spectrum SPF 45
2. $$ PCA Sheer Tint Broad Spectrum SPF 45 with CoQ10
3. $$ TIZO Ultra Zinc Body and Face Sunscreen SPF 40

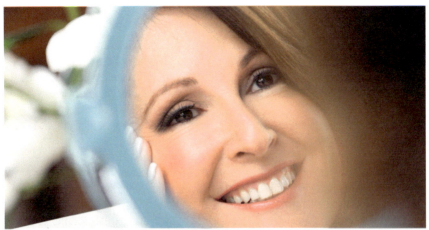

PART II—ANTI-AGING THERAPIES FOR SKIN THAT STANDS THE TEST OF TIME

Increasing scientific knowledge and advances in medical technology have extended our lifespan and have had a profound impact the way we age. From synthetic blood to artificial retinas, innovations emerge every day that have the power to mitigate many of the physical limitations and chronic diseases of aging. If these advances allow us to live longer and feel younger, we very rightly want them to help us look younger too!

Lest you assume the quest for ageless skin is a modern preoccupation, I should point out that the use of medicinal plants for personal care and beauty stems from many ancient traditions—Asian, Native American, aboriginal, and others. These botanical applications are grounded in a firm belief that our bodies must be in harmony with our minds and with our environments, and they work compatibly with other holistic lifestyle therapies.

WHAT CAUSES AGING?

There are many theories of aging, but one of particular relevance to skin health and longevity is the "inflammation theory of aging." The Inflammation Theory of Aging asserts that the single greatest precipitator of aging and age-related diseases is inflammation caused by oxidative (or free radical) stress and damage. Although it is still not clear whether aging causes inflammation or inflammation causes aging . . . or both . . . many medical doctors see inflammation, which occurs on a cellular level, as the precursor to many of our modern health conditions, including heart disease, Alzheimer's and, yes, even skin issues, from sagging skin to wrinkles to lesions to certain kinds of cancers.

INFLAMMATION AND YOUR SKIN

The physical signs of aging can sometimes take us by surprise. Remember when you noticed your first gray hair? Those fine lines that seemed to show up out of the blue one day were, in fact, gradually developing day after day, year after year. Some signs of skin aging are quite natural and can be expected, but others are premature and are often accelerated by our lifestyle choices.

INTRINSIC AGING

Intrinsic aging is a normal phenomenon related to the passage of time and natural aging processes. To some degree it is related to our genes, but not entirely. More and more, science bears out that even our DNA can be manipulated by lifestyle. What are the "normal" things one might expect to see happen to our skin through the normal aging process?

- Skin that is still smooth and unblemished, but now begins to show mild thinning, along with slightly less collagen, which gives skin its firmness and shape.

- Slower cell "turnover" time. Skin cells replace themselves about every 20 days in young adults and approximately every 30 days in older adults. This explains the longer healing times in older patients after dermabrasion or laser resurfacing. This, along with less effective desquamation (natural shedding of surface cells) can result in the "dull" appearance we often see with older skin.

- Facial movement lines (sometimes called laugh lines or worry lines) which start to show up in your 40s and 50s on the forehead, above the nose, and around the mouth and eyes.

EXTRINSIC AGING

Extrinsic aging is often caused by lifestyle factors that contribute to an inflammatory condition in the body, resulting in premature aging. These factors are considered to be responsible for 80% of the skin aging process.

- Sun exposure—One of the primary causes of skin damage is sun exposure. The sun's ultraviolet (UV) light breaks down the elastin in skin, causing it to stretch, sag, wrinkle and become blotchy. It can also lead to skin cancer. The common misperception is that skin cancer from the sun happens only to the very old. Each year a million Americans will develop a skin cancer by age 65.
- Smoking
- Excessive alcohol
- Poor diet, nutritional deficiencies
- Hormone deficiencies—As we age, our skin becomes thinner and there is a decline in collagen. Studies show that this occurs at a greater rate during the first few years after menopause.
- Stress

THESE FACTORS CAN LEAD TO THE FOLLOWING SKIN CONDITIONS AND FUTURE HEALTH CONCERNS:
— Thin, "crepey" skin with fine lines and wrinkles
— Dry or roughened skin
— Pigmented lesions such as freckles, lentigines (brown spots), patchy hyperpigmentation and depigmentation (pale or white spots)

- Loss of tone and elasticity, especially around the eyes, cheeks and jawline (due to lowered levels of collagen, elastin and glycosaminoglycan, one of which is hyaluronic acid)
- Increased skin fragility and areas of purpura (rashes of purple spots caused by blood vessel weakness)
- Benign lesions such as keratoses, spider veins, skin tags (moles), and cherry angiomas
- Greater susceptibility to bruising due to decreased elasticity
- Skin cancers
- Greater vulnerability to cold sore outbreaks

WHAT YOU CAN DO NOW FOR RADIANT SKIN AND LIFELONG VITALITY

REDUCE INFLAMMATION
- Eat a "clean" diet. (See dietary recommendations on page 8)
- Manage stress. Stress can destroy skin structures, as well as joints, brain cells, and arteries.
- Take fish oil daily for Omega-3 "essential" fatty acids. These help to fortify the skin, to support our arteries and joints, and to build our immune defenses.

PROTECT YOURSELF FROM UV DAMAGE
- Wear protective sunscreens. Use only zinc or titanium oxide based sunscreens. (See page X for recommended products.)
- Wear sun protective clothing. This is important, especially when you expect to be outdoors with prolonged exposure, as when hiking, playing tennis or golf, swimming, sailing, etc. See these websites for good sun protective clothing:
    www.Sunprecautions.com
    www.Solartex.com
    www.Coolibar.com

EXPLORE CUTTING-EDGE ANTI-AGING PRODUCTS
The products listed below are often referred to as "actives," as they can actually change the condition of your skin.

- HYDROXYACIDS AND RETINOIDS. I recommend these to older patients because they "speed up" the cell cycle, consequently leading to faster healing times and enhanced skin "brightness."
- ORAL AND TOPICAL ANTIOXIDANTS. Topical antioxidants help protect your skin from the damage caused by UV light and other environmental stressors known to cause skin damage (age spots, sagging skin, broken vessels and skin cancers) including air pollution, ozone and cigarette smoke. Topical antioxidants include various acids (such as alpha hydroxy acid and ferulic acid) and vitamins (such as A, C, D and E). These popular anti-aging remedies are now also being studied as "chemopreventative" options to prevent skin cancer. Apply these creams and serums to the skin in the morning after cleansing and before applying moisturizers and sunscreens.

- TOPICAL RETINOIDS. Topical agents (such as tretinoin) and in-office procedures focus on "resurfacing" the upper layers of skin. The goal is to remove the damaged epidermis and, in some cases, dermis, and allow them to be replaced with remodeled skin layers. Although there are many treatments available for prematurely aged skin, prevention is still paramount.

BALANCE YOUR HORMONES
- MINERAL SUPPLEMENTATION. One easy, safe, and less invasive way to balance your hormones is through mineral supplementation. Most Americans are woefully deficient in critical minerals such as potassium, selenium, zinc, and magnesium, which support energy needs, emotional balance, and sleep. Many people suffering from adrenal fatigue and poor thyroid function can address these issues with a good mineral supplement.

- BIOIDENTICAL HRT. One clinical study showed that women on HRT had a skin collagen content that was 48% higher than that of women not on HRT. It is important to differentiate between types of HRT. Conjugated equine estrogen and progestin, which are marketed under brand names such as Premarin, have been linked to greater risk of breast cancer. However, a combination of estradiol and progesterone, which are bioidentical, has not. In fact, studies show that this type of HRT actually lowers the risk of breast cancer. The best time to begin HRT is before and during menopause. It will help keep your skin healthy (as well as your heart, arteries, and bones).

ACCENTUATE THE POSITIVE
Sometimes the easiest remedies are the simplest. Take a look at these inside "tricks of the trade" that take very little effort and can make a big difference in the naturalness and beauty of your appearance from day to day:

- AVOID THICK FOUNDATIONS that can accumulate in the lines and accentuate them.
- USE LIP PLUMPING GLOSS OR LIPSTICK. This will smooth out lip wrinkles and lines.
- DUST WITH A FINE MINERAL "SPARKLE" powder after applying a moisturizing foundation to make dull skin appear bright.
- DON'T STAY IN BED TOO LONG. Once you get your necessary 7–8 hours of restorative sleep, get up. This can help prevent puffy eyes.
- Exercise. Thirty minutes of aerobic exercise will uplift your face, resulting in rosy cheeks and shiny eyes. Other kinds of exercise—such as yoga—stimulate the lymph glands, which is detoxifying.
- TRY MICRODERMABRASION THERAPY, along with a hydrating facial. Microdermabrasion therapy, which uses a minimally abrasive instrument to gently sand your skin, removes the thicker outer layer. It requires no downtime and is often used to treat discoloration, sun damage or stretch marks. It will temporarily help skin look plumper and allow makeup to "go on better."

- CONSIDER A WEEKEND LASER PEEL. Laser peels direct short, concentrated pulsating beams of light at irregular skin, precisely removing skin layer by layer. It can brighten the skin for many weeks after only a few days of downtime (flaking and peeling).

- INJECTIONS OF BOTULINUM TOXIN (BOTOX COSMETIC, DYSPORT, XEOMIN) for frown lines, forehead lines and crow's feet. This lasts 3 to 4 months and, if used regularly, can keep wrinkles in these areas at bay. Note: Always have a qualified practitioner perform this procedure.

THOSE LITTLE EXTRAS

- MASSAGE—We all know the benefits of massage to a sore and stressed body. But it has many skin benefits as well. Because it stimulates blood flow and promotes lymphatic drainage (moving toxins out of cells), it can vitalize a dull complexion. In fact, facial massage can also help to plump slack skin, while also tightening the flesh under the chin to make it firmer. I recommend a monthly facial massage performed by a trained medical aesthetician. It's best not to do this at home, because the lymphatic flow patterns are very specific and require training to understand. Facial massage is especially effective when combined with a calming and hydrating oatmeal and honey mixture.
- STEAM ROOMS AND SAUNAS—Steam rooms and saunas are excellent for detoxifying the skin and body, providing a natural, deep cleansing. They accelerate the body's natural mechanisms (circulation and sweating) for ridding itself of impurities, and some doctors even claim they help to increase collagen. They are also very relaxing and great for alleviating stress. However, they can also over-dry the skin. Don't use them frequently or stay in them for too long (no more than about 15–20 minutes). Always hydrate well and moisturize the skin afterwards.
- MASKS—Masks can be very beneficial to the skin and are often used as spa treatments. Clay masks are more of a drying agent, so would work better for oily, acne-prone skin. Mud masks have more of a hydrating quality, cleansing the skin of impurities, improving circulation, and moisturizing at a deep level. Alba Hawaiian Facial Mask, with Papaya Enzyme, Laura Mercier Deep Cleansing Mask, and Jan Marini Factor A Plus Mask are three masks that I recommend to my clients.

> As you can see, many skin issues are specific (but not inevitable) to aging, and are often a result of a chronic inflammatory condition in the body. In the next chapter we'll take a closer look at one of these skin problems—cold sores—a common health concern that almost everyone has experienced at some point in their lives. It can cause embarrassment and be symptomatic of deeper health issues but, as with many skin conditions, it is also easily preventable and highly treatable through diet and lifestyle.

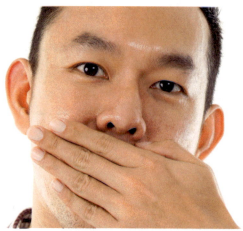

PART III—COLD SORE PREVENTION & IMMUNE SYSTEM SUPPORT

Your skin is a mirror or signpost of what is going wrong (or right) elsewhere in your body. Unhealthy skin is often a reflection of something more serious taking place at a systemic level, such as inflammation, which compromises your immunity and makes you vulnerable to viruses. One of the more common signs of a compromised immune system is cold sores—also known as the herpes simplex virus. Perhaps as much as 2/3rds of the U.S. population may harbor the cold sore herpes virus. Although many of us carry the virus around with us all our lives, we may never experience an outbreak or only experience one when our bodies are weakened.

COLD SORES—HERPES SIMPLEX (HSV-1)

The herpes virus is not new. It's been around for centuries. The Ancient Greek scholar Hippocrates documented several cases, referring to the condition as "herpein," which means "to crawl" or "to creep" because of the spreading nature of herpes skin lesions. There are literally more than 80 different types of herpes viruses—in fact, chicken pox and shingles are considered herpes viruses—but only about 10% of these viruses affect humans.

The most common type of the herpes simplex virus is HSV-1, which only affects the mouth and lips, resulting in blisters commonly known as "cold sores" or "fever blisters." It would be hard to find anyone who hasn't experienced a cold sore at one time or another, and they often surface during or after an illness when the immune system is compromised.

Although medical doctors will tell you that the virus stays with you for life, there are a number of factors that can keep it at bay so that you avoid future outbreaks. In this section, we provide a few guidelines for building a strong immune system to decrease or prevent the likelihood of an outbreak or to help you heal quickly if one should happen.

COLD SORE TRIGGERS

Cold sores are typically spread from skin-to-skin contact, such as kissing, with an infected person, but it is also possible to get them from shared household items, such as razors, towels, cups and glasses or eating utensils, if the person with the virus has an active lesion (outbreak). Cold sore outbreaks are the result of a compromised immune system and, as I've mentioned, these factors are often tied to lifestyle choices and diet. Here are a few of the factors that can lead to an outbreak:

- Stress
- UV radiation from too much sun exposure
- Extreme heat and cold
- An acidic environment in the gut, which can cause an overpopulation of unhealthy gut microflora (bacteria), resulting in candida and other yeast-related problems
- Sugar
- Processed and fortified foods, trans fats, fast foods, etc.
- A low-grade infection somewhere else in the body. This is why cold sores will often surface following a high fever.
- Some women report that their menstrual cycle will trigger an outbreak. This is why when a woman is menstruating she should get plenty of rest, eat properly, and reduce stress.
- Foods (See below.)

BOOSTING THE IMMUNE SYSTEM AND YOUR HEALING PROCESS

Remember, it is important to not just avoid the foods and behaviors that are known to accelerate viral replication and outbreak, but to embrace a healthy regimen that supports your immune system and builds strength on a daily basis. This includes the following lifestyle habits:

- Hydrate properly
- Exercise regularly
- Choose foods that support immunity
- Consume alcohol at a minimum
- Get a full night's sleep
- Practice relaxation techniques, such as deep breathing or meditation
- Maintain optimum weight
- Wash your hands frequently
- Avoid eating molding food—Many wheat products contain mold, from crackers to cookies to bread. Nuts, rice and syrups can also be contaminated with mold.

FOODS TO CHOOSE, FOODS TO LOSE

Many people don't realize that there are everyday foods that can, and often do, trigger outbreaks.

There are two amino acids in foods that are central to understanding how a herpes condition occurs and how it can be prevented—arginine and lysine.

Neither of these amino acids is inherently unhealthy for the body. But when it comes to cold sores, the issue is an over-abundance of arginine foods along with a shortage of lysine foods. So, in addition to eliminating or reducing high arginine/low lysine foods, you should incorporate more lysine foods in your diet. Lysine helps to push arginine out of your body's cells, preventing the virus from making copies of itself.

LOSE

Those who suffer from the herpes simplex virus should avoid excess consumption of high arginine/low lysine foods such as nuts, chocolate, wheat products, seeds, soy, etc. Supplementing with L-Lysine can be very helpful (see "Supplements" below).

In addition, cold sore sufferers should avoid foods that are overly acidic. An acidic condition in the body is known to weaken the immune system, making you more susceptible to infections and viruses like herpes. An acidic condition can result from too much sugar, food additives, alcohol, processed foods, refined carbs, trans fats, artificial sweeteners, caffeine and too much red meat.

CHOOSE
HIGH-LYSINE FOODS

In addition to avoiding high arginine foods, it is critical to simultaneously choose foods high in lysine. These include cruciferous vegetables such as broccoli, Brussels sprouts, cabbage, cauliflower, kale, collard greens, turnips, bok choy, and arugula, etc.

Although certain fruits are high in lysine, be careful not to consume too much, as they contain sugar. These sugars may be natural, but they will still contribute to an acidic condition in the body. For promoting an alkaline gut environment vs. acidic, consider sour fruits, such as lemons and limes, and berries such as cranberry and elderberry. If you drink fruit juices, make sure there is no added sugar.

YOGURT

Another good choice is yogurt. This has one of the highest amounts of lysine of any food around, and it also contains beneficial bacterial strains that restore the microflora in your gut to build energy and resist disease. Be sure to select yogurt that doesn't contain sugar. Greek yogurts such as FAGE, Stonyfield Organic Greek, and Wallaby Organic Greek are excellent choices.

SPICES AND HERBS THAT HAVE ANTI-MICROBIAL PROPERTIES
- Ginger
- Oregano
- Turmeric
- Clove
- Cinnamon
- Liquorice Root

PREBIOTICS
- Garlic
- Leeks
- Onions
- Artichokes
- Horseradish
- Supplements, such as inulin or FOS (which preferentially ferments inulin)

TEAS
- Green tea—Has been clinically shown to inhibit influenza and to be a supportive anti-viral remedy against herpes.
- Echinacea—Supports the immune system and also has been proven to reduce the severity and duration of viral infections.
- Elderberry—A double blind trial showed elderberry extract's ability to reduce symptoms of influenza and speed recovery. It also showed elderberry's ability to enhance immune response with higher levels of antibodies in the blood. It is believed to inhibit a virus's ability to penetrate healthy cells and to protect cells with powerful antioxidants. Elderberry has also been shown to inhibit replication in four strains of herpes viruses.
- Calendula—The calendula flower promotes skin healing and has anti-inflammatory and antimicrobial properties.

HEALTHY OILS
And finally, make sure you are cooking with healthy oils, such as extra virgin olive oil or coconut oil. Don't overheat your oils or allow them to turn rancid. It is best to steam your vegetables in pure spring water or sauté them in olive oil on low heat or to use these oils uncooked in dressings and dips.

I recommend you get at least a teaspoon or two of coconut oil everyday. Why? Because coconut oil contains something called medium chain fatty acids—lauric acid and caprylic acid, which have antiviral, antifungal, and antibacterial properties that help defend against everything from yeast infections to hepatitis C to herpes.

VITAMINS AND OTHER SUPPLEMENTS FOR IMMUNE SUPPORT
- L-LYSINE (Take 500–1,250 milligrams a day on an empty stomach.)—This amino acid has been used in the treatment of cold sores and is found in many protein foods such as yogurt, meat, milk, and beans. Unfortunately, it loses a lot of its bioavailability when it is cooked, which makes supplementation critical.

> The most important thing to remember about preventing and treating cold sores is to "lose" foods that are high in arginine and "choose" foods that are high in lysine instead.from UV damage and help prevent the appearance of wrinkles, fine lines, and skin discolorations.

- VITAMIN D3 (2000–5000 IU daily)—
People who have a deficiency in Vitamin D are more likely to develop cold sores. Note: it's best to have your doctor check your levels. Anything under "50ng/ml" is considered less than required for optimal health.

- **VITAMIN C (1–3g/daily)**—This multipurpose vitamin increases white blood cells and antibodies and builds collagen.
ZINC (25–50mg/daily)—This immune system supporter can also be found in foods such as mushrooms, collard greens, squash and lamb.

- **SELENIUM (100–300mg/daily)**—This trace mineral helps to protect against infection, while deficiencies have been linked to an increased susceptibility to viruses.
- **BEE PROPOLIS (50–150 mg daily)**—Propolis, like honey, is a product that bees make—a sticky glue-like substance they use to patch holes and seal cracks in their hives. It is known to have many health benefits, including antimicrobial properties that make it an excellent defense against viruses and bacteria. It also inhibits infections from occurring, including yeast infections (candida).
- **MUSHROOMS SUCH AS GANODERMA LUCIDUM** (available in pill form or as a tea). More commonly known as reishi or lingzhi, Ganoderma has an alkalizing and oxygenating effect on the body. It is an excellent skin remedy, as it is known to improve skin texture, inhibit free radicals, and rejuvenate body tissues and cells. It also has anti-inflammatory and anti-viral properties, and is one of nature's greatest immune system boosters.

Before reading this booklet, you may have thought of your skin as something that simply takes care of itself. I hope that now you will be encouraged to think of your skin as something not to be neglected, but to nurture and care for. As with other critical organs in the body, your skin must be supported with diet, targeted supplementation, and healthy daily rituals. No matter what your age, you have the power to change your health in ways that enhance the way you look and feel.

If you have questions, please contact me at:

Laura Ellis MD Skin Care & Vein Centre, PLLC
30 Town Square Blvd, Suite 218
Asheville, NC 28803

828.684.1212
www.lauraellismd.com | www.medage.com

FAQs

1. I'D LIKE TO SIMPLIFY MY SKIN CARE ROUTINE. WHAT ARE THE 5 MOST IMPORTANT PRODUCTS YOU SUGGEST I USE?

- Non soap cleanser—use twice daily, in the morning and evening
- Sunscreen—every day
- Tretinoin (Retin A)—apply after cleansing every evening. There are over-the-counter preparations or a stronger version that can be prescribed by your doctor, usually in a 0.1–0.05% cream. Those with sensitive skin may find that this causes skin dryness, redness or flaking. If so, begin with three evenings per week. Then, after two weeks, gradually increase to every night.
- Moisturizer—every day and night
- Emollient eye cream

2. SHOULD I USE BENZOYL PEROXIDE?

No. Benzoyl peroxide kills bacteria by generating free radicals and free radicals are known to lead to accelerated aging of the skin. When applied at the same time as topical tretinoin, benzoyl peroxide can denature (break down) the tretinoin and reduce its effectiveness.

3. WHICH SUNSCREENS OFFER THE BEST PROTECTION?

First, select a broad spectrum sunscreen that blocks both UVA and UVB. In particular, choose a sunscreen that includes a good level (4% to 5%) of zinc oxide (also called micronized zinc or Z-cote), or titanium dioxide, or Parsol 1789 (also called avobenzone) or Mexoryl (also called ecamsule) among the list of active ingredients.

Second, choose a sunscreen with a **SPF 20** rating or higher – this is the minimum level now recommended by most dermatologists.

Third, determine the activity you will be doing for the day and apply a product that will meet the task, e.g. water activities mean you should use a waterproof sunscreen.

Fourth, always choose a sunscreen that feels good on your skin – so you will be comfortable wearing it every day. Once you have found a sunscreen or several that meet these four needs, use it regularly and properly and it will provide excellent sun protection.

4. HOW SHOULD SUNSCREEN BE APPLIED?

Sunscreens do not work without proper application, nor will they work for longer than two hours without reapplication.

First, apply sunscreen 20 minutes before going outside to allow it time to penetrate or bind to the skin.

Second, you need to use an adequate amount. If you under apply you are likely to get burned. This is probably the most common mistake made by sunscreen users. The recommended level is 2 mg sunscreen/square cm skin. For the average adult needing coverage at the beach, this means using a shot glass full of sunscreen per application.

Third, even if the label says "all day protection" you should reapply every two hours while outside until sunset. The term "very water resistant" means one must reapply every 90 minutes when swimming, while "water resistant" means one must reapply every 40 minutes when swimming.

Fourth, do not use old sunscreen. Check the expiration date and throw away old sunscreens. Active ingredients lose their potency over time.

5. WHAT IF I ALREADY HAVE SUN DAMAGE?

Many people over the age of 40 have skin that is significantly damaged from the sun. Fortunately, those who are younger know more about the dangers of tanning and have had access to better sun protection products than previous generations. For sun damaged skin:

- Consult with an experienced cosmetic physician. Certain cosmeceutical products such as skin hydrators (see moisturizer suggestions on page 12) can be used at home.
- There also are in-office procedures that enhance absorption of hydrators, such as hyaluronic acid, by "driving" them through the surface of the skin. The Hydrafacial system is a good example.
- A series of micro needling procedures can encourage new collagen growth especially when combined with PRP (platelet rich plasma) collected directly from the patient, and stem cells (from amniotic fluid) collected from live, healthy Cesarean births and purchased from a medical tissue bank.
- Laser skin resurfacing can be used as a "weekend peel" (light resurfacing with only 2–3 days downtime consisting of flaking skin), or as a full, deep resurfacing for extremely sun damaged skin (with a 7–10 day healing period consisting of redness, swelling, extreme peeling and even some oozing).

6. ARE THERE ANY COLD SORE OUTBREAK TRIGGERS THAT ARE NOT COMMONLY KNOWN OR ADDRESSED?

Yes, many individuals seem to have certain sensitivities to uncommon triggers, in addition to the common ones, such as stress, UV sunlight and chocolate and nuts. First, as we mentioned, it's the arginine in the chocolate and nuts that can be a problem, especially if it overpowers the lysine in your system. That's why it's best to take L-lysine daily, as a supplement. Keep in mind that many performance enhancing supplements, powders, and drinks for weekend warriors, body builders, etc. are high in arginine. Some people find that certain enzymes, such as the bromelain found in pineapple, can also trigger an outbreak, especially if they're under stress or their immune system is weakened. That's why a good daily immune boosting supplement may also be helpful to reduce the frequency and/or severity of outbreaks.

7. DOES THE HSV-1 VIRUS THAT'S RESPONSIBLE FOR COLD SORES ONLY CAUSE OUTBREAKS AROUND THE FACE?

The HSV-1 cold sore virus can also contribute to outbreaks around the genital area. This is why it's extremely important to not touch this area with hands that may have had contact with a facial cold sore. In fact, it's estimated that up to 40% of genital herpes cases were actually caused by the HSV-1 cold sore virus.

Made in the USA
Columbia, SC
09 July 2024